Simplified Solution Approach To MYASTHENIA GRAVIS

Unlocking Inner Strength: A Comprehensive Guide to Overcoming Neuromuscular Challenges and Reclaiming Vitality

Dr QUENTIN GLYN

Table Of Contents

CHAPTER ONE
Myasthenia Gravis

Muscle weakness and exhaustion are hallmarks of the chronic autoimmune neuromuscular disease known as myasthenia gravis (MG). The illness develops when the body's immune system unintentionally targets the neuromuscular junction, which connects muscles and nerve signals. This causes a breakdown in the nerve-muscle transmission, which leads to weakness and exhaustion, especially in the muscles controlling the motions of the eyes, mouth, swallowing, chewing, and limbs.

Myasthenia gravis management presents several difficulties that need a comprehensive approach to solutions in order to improve the quality of life for those afflicted. Simplifying the approach is crucial to optimizing patient outcomes, streamlining treatment, and reducing the complexity involved in managing this illness.

A Synopsis Of Myasthenia Gravis:

Comprehending the complexities of Myasthenia Gravis is essential to creating a streamlined remedy strategy that works. Key characteristics of MG consist of:

Autoimmune Nature: Myasthenia Gravis (MG) is an autoimmune illness in which the body's immune system generates antibodies directed against the acetylcholine receptors on muscle cells. This results in a disruption of nerve-muscle transmission.

Variable Symptoms: There may be a significant range of MG symptoms from person to person. Muscle weakness, double vision, difficulties swallowing, and breathing problems are common symptoms. There may be phases of aggravation and remission in the intensity of the symptoms.

Difficulties in Diagnosing: Because MG symptoms may vary widely and overlap with other neurological disorders, diagnosing MG can be difficult. A combination of clinical assessment, neurophysiological testing, and antibody assays is often used to get an accurate diagnosis.

Options for Treatment: Although there isn't a cure for MG, there are a number of treatments that try to control symptoms and enhance neuromuscular function. These might include immunosuppressive medicines and acetylcholinesterase inhibitors, as well as, in some situations, surgery.

Importance Of A Simplified Approach To Solutions:

It is essential to use a streamlined solution approach for several reasons:

Improved Patient Compliance: Patients' adherence to treatment plans is increased when MG is easier to control. Overwhelming complex treatment regimens might cause non-adherence. Simplifying treatments increases the likelihood that patients will adhere to their treatment plans, which improves results.

Optimized Healthcare Resources: The best utilization of healthcare resources is achieved via streamlining MG management. This is particularly crucial for those with chronic illnesses who may need continuous care. Healthcare systems are less burdened when resources are allocated efficiently, ensuring that patients get timely and appropriate treatments.

Better Quality of Life: Improving the lives of those impacted by MG is the main objective of the condition's management. Patients may more easily manage the difficulties brought on by MG when a more straightforward approach lessens the physical and psychological strain on them.

Patient education and assistance may be made more accessible by using a more straightforward approach. Giving patients information that is easy to grasp gives them the ability to actively engage in their treatment. As a result, they become more confident and in charge of their condition management.

Multidisciplinary Collaboration: Healthcare experts from many disciplines collaborate more when things are simplified. A multidisciplinary approach guarantees that the treatment plan takes into account the physical, psychological, and social components of MG.

To sum up, a more straightforward approach to treating Myasthenia Gravis is essential for maximizing patient care, making sure that resources are used effectively, and eventually raising the standard of living for those who suffer from this difficult autoimmune neuromuscular disease. For a strategy like this to be successful in streamlining therapies and improving the efficacy of MG management regimens, patients, researchers, and healthcare professionals must work together.

CHAPTER TWO

Knowledge Of Myasthenia Gravis

Let's dissect the ideas around Myasthenia Gravis (MG) into three primary categories: Pathophysiology, Etiology and Risk Factors, and Definition and Classification.

Meaning And Categorization:

Muscle weakness and exhaustion are hallmarks of the chronic autoimmune neuromuscular disease known as myasthenia gravis (MG). The creation of antibodies that target and disrupt the function of acetylcholine receptors (AChR) at the neuromuscular junction, resulting in impaired nerve-muscle communication, is a characteristic of myasthenia gravis (MG). This may cause a variety of muscle groups, including those that govern swallowing, facial expressions, and limb motions, to become weaker, particularly during repeated movements.

Grouping:

Multiple muscle groups, including those that regulate the eyes, face, limbs, and respiratory system, are affected by generalized myopathy.

Ocular MG: Ptosis (drooping eyelids) and diplopia (double vision) are mostly caused by this condition, which affects the muscles that govern eye movements.

Mild MG: Minimal influence on day-to-day activities and limited muscle involvement.

Severe MG: Causes significant muscular weakness and may make it difficult to carry out essential tasks like breathing.

Causes And Precursors:

Etiology: Although the precise etiology of MG is unknown, an autoimmune illness is thought to be the likely culprit. When an autoimmune disease occurs, the body's own tissues are unintentionally targeted and attacked by the immune system. The immune system attacks the AChR in MG because it is essential for signal transmission from the nerves to the muscles.

Gender and Age: Although MG may strike anybody at any age, it is more frequent in males over 60 and women under 40.

Thymus organ Abnormalities: MG patients often have anomalies in the thymus, an organ that is important in the immune system. MG is linked to thymic tumors, sometimes referred to as thymomas, an enlarged thymus, or hyperplasia.

Hereditary Factors: Since MG may run in families, there may be a hereditary component to the condition.

Other Autoimmune Diseases: People who suffer from lupus or rheumatoid arthritis, for example, maybe more susceptible to getting MG.

Pathophysiology Of Grave Myasthenia:

Impairment of the neuromuscular junction:

Normal Transmission: Acetylcholine (ACh) is released at the neuromuscular junction as nerve impulses travel along nerve fibers.

Muscle contraction results from the binding of ACh to AChR on the muscle cell membrane.

Production of Antibodies: The body creates antibodies that attack and degrade AChR, primarily immunoglobulin G, or IgG.

Reduced Nerve Signal Transmission: Antibodies obstruct or eliminate AChR, which lowers the transmission efficiency of nerve signals.

Weakened Signals Cause Muscular Weakness and Fatigue: Weakened signals cause muscular weakness, particularly with repeated usage. muscular exhaustion over time may cause symptoms including drooping eyes, trouble swallowing, and widespread muscular weakness.

Immunosuppressive therapy to control the immunological response, medicines to enhance neuromuscular transmission, and sometimes, surgery to correct thymus anomalies are all common components of treatment plans. Effective management of MG requires multidisciplinary treatment including immunologists, neurologists, and other medical specialists, as well as routine medical monitoring.

CHAPTER THREE
Presentation Of Clinical Data

The neuromuscular condition known as myasthenia gravis (MG) is characterized by weariness and muscle weakness. The illness is brought on by a breakdown in the nerve-muscle communication system, which makes it difficult to regulate voluntary muscle movements.

Individual differences may be seen in the clinical presentation of MG, and successful care requires a thorough knowledge of the symptoms, diagnosis, and impact on day-to-day functioning.

Indices And Outward Signs:

1. Weakness of Muscles:

• Muscle weakness is one of the main symptoms, usually originating in the face and neck.

• Patients often struggle with tasks involving fine motor skills, such as eating, smiling, or holding a pen.

2. Diplopia with Ptosis:

• Drooping of the eyelids, or ptosis, is a typical early sign.

Diplopia, or double vision, may happen when the muscles that govern eye movement become weak.

3. Weary:

• A defining trait of MG is a weakness that usually becomes worse with exercise and gets better with rest.

• Patients may experience greater tiredness all day long, particularly after engaging in repeated motions.

4. Symptoms of the bulge:

Slurred speech and dysphagia (difficulty swallowing) may be caused by the weakening of the muscles that perform these tasks.

5. Respiratory Participation:

• Breathlessness and respiratory discomfort may result from severe instances that impair the respiratory muscles.

Differential Diagnosis And Diagnosis:

1. Clinical Assessment:

• Gathering information on the beginning and development of symptoms.

• A physical examination that highlights the involvement of certain muscle groups and muscular strength.

2. Exams Neurological:

• Pay close attention to limb weakness, face muscle strength, and eye motions.

• Electromyography and repetitive nerve stimulation tests are two methods for evaluating neuromuscular transmission.

3. Blood Examinations:

• The diagnosis is confirmed by serological testing, which includes acetylcholine receptor (AChR) and muscle-specific kinase (MuSK) antibodies.

4. Imaging Research:

• Thymoma, a condition linked to MG, may be ruled out using imaging methods such as CT or MRI scans.

Diagnostic Differentiation:

• Myasthenic syndrome Lambert-Eaton (LEMS):

• Another autoimmune condition that affects neuromuscular transmission but uses a different kind of antibody.

• Syndrome of Chronic Fatigue:

• Both illnesses often cause fatigue, but MG is characterized by more severe muscular weakness.

Differential Sclerosis:

• While there may be overlap in neurological symptoms, the kind and pattern of weakness vary.

Effects On Day-To-Day Living:

1. Functional Restraints:

• MG may greatly affect day-to-day activity, making even easy chores difficult and draining.

2. Impact on Society and Emotions:

• Anxiety and sadness are two emotional difficulties that might arise from managing a chronic illness.

3. Work and Learning:

• Weakness and fatigue might impair productivity at work or in the classroom, requiring modifications.

4. Life Quality:

• Although MG is a chronic illness, quality of life may be enhanced by sensible management techniques, such as medication and lifestyle modifications.

In summary, Myasthenia Gravis affects several muscle groups and has a substantial influence on day-to-day functioning. It manifests itself via a variety of symptoms.

Improving long-term results and starting the right therapy depends on an early and precise diagnosis. Comprehensive treatment requires a multidisciplinary approach combining immunologists, neurologists, and other medical specialists.

CHAPTER FOUR
Presently Used Treatment Approaches

Muscle weakness and exhaustion are the hallmarks of Myasthenia Gravis (MG), a chronic autoimmune neuromuscular condition usually brought on by antibodies that attack acetylcholine receptors at the neuromuscular junction.

A mix of drugs, immunosuppressive treatments, and, in some situations, surgical procedures like thymectomy are used to control myasthenia gravis. A detailed summary of the available treatment techniques is provided below:

Medications To Alleviate Symptoms:

1. Inhibitors of acetylcholinesterase, such as pyridostigmine:

• By increasing acetylcholine concentration at the neuromuscular junction, these medications strengthen muscles.

• Usually used to treat mild to severe ailments.

Depending on the patient's reaction, the dosage may need to be changed.

2. Immunostimulatory Medication:

• Corticosteroids (Prednisone, for example):

• Applied to lower antibody production and inhibit the immune system.

• Good in managing symptoms, but may have long-term adverse effects.

• IVIG (intravenous immunoglobulin):

• Offers transient relief by preventing the antibodies that cause muscular weakness.

• Often used as a temporary bridging treatment or for acute exacerbations.

• Plasmapheresis, or Plasma Exchange:

• Eliminates dangerous antibodies from the blood, offering momentary yet quick relief.

• Applicable in extreme circumstances or myasthenic crises.

Treatments For Immune Suppression:

1. Azathioprine:

• An agent that spares steroids but suppresses immune cell function by blocking DNA synthesis.

• Takes many months to manifest benefits, but it may help keep remission stable.

2. Mofetil mycophenolate:

• Stunts the growth of lymphocytes, lowering immune system function.

• When other immunosuppressants are not well tolerated, this medication is used.

3. Rituximab:

• A monoclonal antibody that suppresses the synthesis of antibodies by targeting B cells.

• Sometimes successful, particularly when other therapies don't work.

4. Cyclosporine with Tacrolimus:

• Inhibitors of calcineurin that alter T-cell function.

• As an adjuvant to other immunosuppressants or in patients that are not responding well.

As A Form Of Treatment, Thymectomy:

1. Surgical Procedure:

• A thymectomy entails the gland's removal, which is important for producing antibodies.

• May lead to remission or a notable improvement, especially in thymoma patients.

• Patients with widespread MG and those who are younger often have the best results.

2. When to Have a Thymectomy:

When MG first manifests, especially in younger individuals, an early thymectomy is advised.

• Benefits may not always be apparent, and not all MG patients should get it.

3. Minimally Adversarial Methods:

• Robotic-assisted operations or video-assisted thoracoscopic surgery (VATS) may shorten the recuperation period.

Observation And Tailored Care:

1. Frequent Monitoring

• Keeping an eye on side effects from medications, tracking symptoms, and evaluating therapy response.

• Modifying drug doses in accordance with clinical status.

2. Multidisciplinary Method:

• For complete treatment, neurologists, immunologists, and surgeons are involved.

• Working together with occupational and physical therapists to treat symptoms and enhance quality of life.

In summary, a customized strategy is necessary for the management of myasthenia gravis, taking into account the intensity of symptoms, patient characteristics, and therapy response.

Optimizing results for individuals with MG requires a multidisciplinary team, careful monitoring, and individualized therapy.

CHAPTER FIVE
Constraints And Difficulties

Let's talk about the drawbacks and difficulties pertaining to myasthenia gravis (MG), with a specific emphasis on the adverse reactions to existing therapies, the unpredictability of patient reactions, and problems with accessibility and cost.

Side Effects Of Current Treatments:

Acetylcholinesterase inhibitors, immunosuppressive medications, and sometimes thymectomy are among the therapy options often used to control myasthenia gravis. These therapies have disadvantages even if they may be useful in symptom relief.

Immunosuppressive Medications:

A variety of adverse effects, including increased susceptibility to infections, weight gain, mood swings, and loss of bone density, may result from immunosuppressive medications, such as corticosteroids. The long-term use of these drugs has a number of serious health hazards.

Acetylcholinesterase Inhibitors:

These medications may induce gastrointestinal problems, such as nausea, diarrhea, and cramping in the abdomen, but they may also increase muscular strength by improving the transmission between neurons and muscles.

Thymectomy: Although removing the thymus gland may be advantageous for some individuals, there are inherent surgical risks and possible problems associated with this treatment.

Variability In Patient Reaction:

Patients with MG are known to be heterogeneous, displaying a range of severity and therapy responses. This fluctuation may be attributed to many factors:

Disease Severity: There is a spectrum of MG, from moderate to severe, and the best course of therapy may vary depending on the patient.

Thymus Involvement: Individuals with thymic anomalies may react to therapy in various ways, and the particulars of thymus involvement may have an impact on the choice to perform thymectomy.

Individual Immune Response: Patients may experience varying degrees of therapeutic success depending on how their immune systems react to immunosuppressive treatments.

Accessibility And Expense: Two important factors that may have an influence on MG management are the availability of appropriate healthcare and the expense of therapy.

Neurologists or neuromuscular experts are often called upon to provide specialized treatment for patients with MG. In some areas, there may be barriers to accessing these medical personnel, which might result in delayed diagnosis and inadequate treatment.

Cost Of Medications: Certain MG treatments, especially the more recent immunosuppressive ones, have a high price tag. Some patients may find it difficult to follow recommended regimens due to the financial burden of long-term therapy.

Surgical Interventions: Depending on the state of the healthcare system and insurance coverage, a thymectomy, if advised, may not be a surgical operation that is available or cheap for all individuals.

To tackle these issues, current research endeavors to provide more precise, efficacious, and little side effective treatments. Furthermore, in order to guarantee that every person with MG receives the best treatment possible, initiatives to upgrade the healthcare system's infrastructure, raise awareness, and improve costs are essential. Furthermore, patient education and support initiatives may be very important in enabling people to properly manage their conditions.

CHAPTER SIX

The Requirement Of A Simplified Method

Emphasizing Patient-Centered Care And Filling Up Treatment Deficits:

Muscle weakness and exhaustion are hallmarks of the complicated autoimmune disease known as myasthenia gravis (MG). Because MG is so unexpected and varied, managing it may be difficult. It is important to have a streamlined strategy for managing MG for several reasons.

1. MG's Complexity:

The clinical presentations and consequences of myasthenia gravis vary widely, making it a diverse illness. The neuromuscular junction, which is involved in the disruption of nerve and muscle transmission, is the source of the intricacy. It is challenging for patients and healthcare professionals to negotiate the complexities of the condition because of this heterogeneity.

2. Burden of Treatment:

Acetylcholinesterase inhibitors, immunosuppressive drugs, and sometimes invasive procedures like thymectomy are used in conjunction with traditional MG therapy regimens. Patients may have poor adherence and less-than-ideal results as a result of the stress of managing several drugs and possible adverse effects.

3. Effect on Life Quality:

The quality of life of an MG sufferer might be greatly affected by the symptoms' unpredictable nature. By keeping therapy as simple as possible, patients will find it easier to comply with their treatment plans and maintain a higher standard of living.

Justification For A Simplified Approach:

1. Enhanced Compliance:

Higher adherence rates are linked to more straightforward treatment plans. Patients are more likely to comply with their treatment programs when there are fewer drugs, easier dose schedules, and fewer adverse effects. Consequently, this improves the treatment's efficacy.

2. Better Tracking:

Simplifying the process makes patient monitoring easier and more effective. In order to help with the early diagnosis of exacerbations or consequences, healthcare practitioners might concentrate on important markers of disease activity. For treatment regimens to be rapidly adjusted, regular monitoring is essential.

3. Simplified Interaction:

Improved patient-provider communication is fostered by streamlining terminology and descriptions of MG and its treatment. A more cooperative approach to managing illness results from people being empowered to actively engage in their treatment via clear communication.

1. Tailored Care Programs:

Every MG patient has different requirements and preferences, and they are acknowledged in a patient-centered approach. Individualized treatment programs that take into account the patient's interests, preferences, and lifestyle guarantee a more successful and individualized management approach.

2. Cooperative Decision-Making:

Including patients in the choices they make about their care promotes a feeling of empowerment and ownership. Patients are more likely to follow treatment recommendations and express greater satisfaction with their healthcare when they actively engage in choices about their care.

3. Comprehensive Assistance:

A patient-centered approach attends to the whole needs of MG patients, going beyond medical therapy. In order to enhance general well-being, this involves offering resources for mental health assistance, dietary advice, and physical treatment.

Filling In The Treatment Gaps:

1. Knowledge and Consciousness:

It takes a concentrated effort to educate patients and healthcare professionals about MG in order to close treatment gaps. In order to close knowledge gaps and encourage proactive care, it is important to raise awareness of the illness, its symptoms, and the need for prompt and consistent treatment.

2. Obtaining Specialized Care Accessible:

Maximizing treatment success requires guaranteeing access to expert care for MG patients. This entails setting up telemedicine services, educational initiatives, and interdisciplinary clinics to improve the expertise of medical practitioners in treating MG.

3. Investigation and Originality:

In order to find holes in the present treatment procedures and create new, more straightforward solutions, ongoing research and innovation are crucial. Research, physicians, and pharmaceutical corporations working together may provide innovations that meet the changing requirements of MG patients.

In summary, maximizing outcomes in this complex autoimmune condition requires a simple solution approach to Myasthenia Gravis that emphasizes patient-centered care and fills therapeutic gaps. Healthcare professionals may empower patients to better manage their conditions and enhance their overall quality of life by simplifying treatment regimens, improving communication, and encouraging a collaborative approach.

CHAPTER SEVEN

Simplified Solutions That Were Suggested

Muscle weakness and exhaustion are hallmarks of the chronic autoimmune neuromuscular disease known as myasthenia gravis (MG). Although there isn't a cure for MG, there are ways to manage the illness and enhance the lives of those who have it. The condensed solutions that are suggested include integrative methods, supportive treatments, and lifestyle adjustments.

1. Changes In Lifestyle:

a. A well-rounded diet

Make sure to eat a nutritious, well-balanced diet that is high in protein and other nutrients that assist muscular function.

To address any particular dietary issues and customize the diet to meet individual requirements, think about speaking with a nutritionist.

b. Frequent Workout:

Exercises with little impact may help you keep your muscles flexible and strong.

Together with a physical therapist, create a customized workout program that fits the patient's ability.

c. Sufficient Sleep and Rest:

Make getting enough sleep a priority to avoid weariness, which is a typical MG symptom.

Maintain a regular sleep routine to enhance general health.

d. Handling Stress:

Investigate stress-relieving methods like yoga, deep breathing exercises, and meditation.

Since stress may make muscular weakness worse, managing stress can help with MG symptoms.

2. Complementary Medicines:

a. Management of Medication:

Adherence to a neurologist's recommendations about the usage of prescribed drugs, such as immunosuppressants or acetylcholinesterase inhibitors.

Review prescription dosages often and make necessary adjustments.

b. Occupational and Physical Therapy:

Participate in physical therapy to increase muscular strength and range of motion.

If you want to modify your everyday routines and activities to save energy, think about occupational therapy.

c. Helping Tools:

Employ assistive technology to improve movement and lessen the pressure on weakening muscles, such as walkers, canes, or braces.

Collaborate with medical specialists to identify the best assistive technology.

3. Integrative Methods:

a. Both massage and acupuncture:

Investigate alternative treatments such as massage or acupuncture to reduce stress in the muscles and enhance general health.

Make sure professionals with the necessary training and expertise are administering these treatments.

b. Body-Mind Techniques:

Incorporate mind-body exercises to improve your physical and mental health, such as tai chi or qigong.

These exercises could support better muscular control and balance.

c. Supplements for nutrition:

Consult a healthcare provider about the possible advantages of using certain dietary supplements.

Supplements such as omega-3 fatty acids or vitamin D may help some people maintain their general health.

Frequent Observation:

Continue seeing a neurologist for regular check-ups to keep an eye on your MG symptoms and modify your treatment regimen as necessary.

Patient Instruction:

Give MG patients more knowledge about their illness, available treatments, and self-management techniques to empower them.

Social Assistance:

Create a solid support system with friends, family, and support groups to provide both practical and emotional help.

In order to customize these strategies to meet their unique requirements, people with MG must collaborate closely with their healthcare team. The integration of integrative techniques, supportive therapies, and lifestyle adjustments may lead to a more comprehensive and efficient therapy of myasthenia gravis.

CHAPTER EIGHT

Applying A Comprehensive Model Of Care

Muscle weakness and exhaustion are hallmarks of the chronic autoimmune neuromuscular disease known as myasthenia gravis (MG). In order to address the complicated nature of MG and enhance patients' overall well-being, a holistic treatment approach must be put into place. A comprehensive approach emphasizes cooperation, education, and ongoing monitoring while taking into account the patient's social, emotional, and physical needs. Here is a thorough examination of important elements:

1. Healthcare Teams Working Together:

a. Multidisciplinary Method:

Assembling a cooperative team of medical professionals, including immunologists, physical therapists, occupational therapists, and neurologists.

Attend monthly team meetings to talk about therapy modifications, patient progress, and comprehensive care planning.

b. Patient-First Healthcare:

Engaging the patient in the decision-making process guarantees that their desires, objectives, and worries are considered.

Promoting honest dialogue to build understanding and trust between patients and healthcare providers.

C. Integrated Healthcare:

Putting in place a smooth information exchange between healthcare providers to prevent care that is not fragmented.

Making use of electronic health records to improve coordination and provide a thorough summary of the patient's medical background.

2. Patient Empowerment And Education:

a. Understanding Disease:

Teaching patients about the causes, symptoms, and pathophysiology of MG as well as the value of following treatment regimens.

Provide easily available tools for ongoing education, such as pamphlets, internet resources, and support groups.

b. Self-Control Ability:

Providing instruction on how to manage medications, check symptoms on oneself, and spot exacerbation symptoms.

Promoting the development of coping mechanisms to address the psychological and emotional effects of MG.

C. Changes in Lifestyle:

Offering advice on stress reduction, exercise, and diet in order to maximize general health.

Enabling patients to make decisions about lifestyle choices that might affect their condition with knowledge.

3. Observation And Flexible Administration:

a. Frequent Evaluations:

putting into practice a methodical strategy to track the development of the illness by conducting routine laboratory testing, imaging scans, and clinical assessments.

modifying treatment programs in accordance with the patient's changing requirements.

b. Integration of Technology:

using telemedicine to provide remote monitoring and consultations, improving accessibility for those with limited mobility.

use wearable technology and health apps to monitor general health, medication compliance, and symptoms.

C. Plans for Adaptive Care:

creating adaptable care plans that can be changed in response to MG's changing needs.

collaborating with patients to collectively adjust treatment plans as necessary via shared decision-making.

Myasthenia gravis requires a thorough, patient-centered strategy to implement a holistic treatment plan. We can improve treatment quality and overall results for MG patients by encouraging teamwork among healthcare providers, educating patients to take charge of their own health and using adaptive management techniques. In addition to treating the patient's physical symptoms, this holistic approach takes into account their emotional and social needs, enabling them to lead more balanced and satisfying lives even in the face of the difficulties presented by MG.

CHAPTER NINE

Prospects For The Future In Myasthenia Gravis

Muscle weakness and exhaustion are hallmarks of the chronic autoimmune neuromuscular disease known as myasthenia gravis (MG). While the emphasis of present treatments is symptom control, hopeful advancements in upcoming medications, technology advancements, and lobbying initiatives for better resources are all part of the future of MG care.

New Research And Therapies:

1. Immunostimulatory Medication:

• New immunomodulatory treatments are being investigated in order to address the underlying autoimmune response in MG.

• In early clinical studies, biologics that target certain immune pathways, including complement proteins or B cells, are showing promise.

2. Gene and Cell Treatments:

• Advances in gene therapy may give tailored methods to modulate the immune response in MG.

• Research is being done to see if cell-based treatments, such as stem cell transplantation, can balance the immune system again.

3. Precision Health Care:

• The goal of personalized medicine is to customize MG therapy according to each patient's unique immune system and genetic profile.

• To forecast the severity of an illness and direct therapy choices, biomarkers are being discovered.

4. Neuroprotective Techniques:

In an effort to maintain neuromuscular junction function and stop the development of illness, research is looking at neuroprotective medicines.

• Research is being done on neurotrophic factors and other substances that facilitate nerve-muscle connection.

Technological Advancements In The Management Of Groups:

1. Remote monitoring and telemedicine:

• Patients with MG may now get consultations remotely thanks to telemedicine technologies.

• Real-time symptom and medication adherence tracking is made possible by wearable technology and applications.

2. More Advanced Diagnostic Instruments:

• Accurate diagnosis and MG monitoring are made possible by high-resolution imaging methods including magnetic resonance imaging (MRI) and positron emission tomography (PET).

• Research on electrophysiology is still developing, offering comprehensive understanding of the functioning of neuromuscular junctions.

3.Automation and Assistive Technology:

• Exoskeletons and robotics are being investigated to help MG sufferers with everyday tasks and encourage independence.

• People with mobility problems may live better thanks to smart gadgets and home automation technology.

4. Apps for Patient Management:

• Mobile apps that provide details on medication schedules, workout plans, and lifestyle advice help users manage their own health.

• Patients may interact, exchange experiences, and access support networks via these applications.

Promoting Better Resources:

1. Campaigns for Awareness:

• Healthcare organizations and advocacy groups are making a concerted effort to increase public knowledge of MG, shorten the time it takes for a diagnosis, and encourage early intervention.

Campaigns for public awareness are intended to debunk misconceptions about MG and promote mutual understanding across populations.

2. Initiatives for Funding Research:

• The main goal of advocacy work is to get more money for MG research in order to hasten the creation of novel treatments and deepen our knowledge of the condition.

• To advance MG research, cooperation between researchers, pharmaceutical firms, and patient advocacy organizations is crucial.

3. Advocating for Health Policy:

• Advocacy organizations are essential in promoting laws that provide fair access to MG therapies and related services.

• The goal is to persuade healthcare policymakers to give rare illnesses top priority and provide MG sufferers with all-encompassing treatment.

4. Empowerment of Patients:

• One of the main advocacy objectives is to provide people with information about their disease and available treatments.

• Patient advocacy organizations strive to give MG sufferers a say in the formulation of healthcare policies and decision-making processes.

In conclusion, with developments in advocacy, technology, and medicines, the management of Myasthenia Gravis has a bright future ahead of it. The combined efforts of medical professionals, researchers, patients, and advocacy organizations will help to improve the quality of life for those with MG as long as science and technology continue to advance.

Conclusion

The conclusion offers a synopsis and a last reflection on the subject. When it comes to Myasthenia Gravis (MG), it is imperative to stress the value of an all-encompassing, patient-centered approach. Here, the emphasis should be on how crucial it is to combine different tactics and therapies in order to properly manage the illness. Additionally, you may want to emphasize the continuing nature of managing MG and the need for ongoing care and adaptation.

Summary Of Important Points:

Go over the primary ideas that were covered in the body of your work again. This may involve elements like:

Comprehending MG:

Give a brief recap of MG's symptoms, highlighting its autoimmune origins and effects on neuromuscular transmission.

Diagnostic Difficulties:

Review the difficulties in identifying MG because of its wide range of symptoms and the need of a comprehensive evaluation by medical specialists.

Methods of Treatment:

List the many forms of therapy, such as thymectomy, medicine, and supportive treatments.

A Look at Lifestyle:

Stress the need to change one's lifestyle to control MG symptoms, including stress reduction, getting enough sleep, and eating a healthy diet.

Promotion of a Holistic Strategy:

The need to treat the patient holistically—addressing both the physical and emotional elements of living with MG—is emphasized in this section, which is critical.

Empowerment of Patients:

Motivate patients to take an active role in their care by being aware of their health, following their treatment regimens, and successfully interacting with medical professionals.

Emotional Health:

Draw attention to how MG affects mental health and emphasize how crucial emotional wellness is. Promote the use of therapy, support groups, and other tools that may provide psychological assistance.

Exercise and Diet:

Stress the need to lead a healthy lifestyle in the management of MG. A healthy diet and regular exercise may improve general well-being and perhaps lessen the symptoms of MG.

An Appeal For Better Treatment Of Myasthenia Gravis:

Inspire action for improved MG care on a larger scale in this part.

Lobbying:

Promote the financing of MG research and campaigning for MG awareness. Stress how critical it is that the general population comprehends and supports people who are living with MG.

Collaboration between healthcare providers:

Encourage more cooperation between medical professionals, researchers, and experts in order to exchange ideas, create novel therapies, and raise the standard of care for patients with MG.

Instruction and Practice:

Encourage continuing education and training for medical staff members so they may remain informed about the most recent developments in MG management. Improved treatment plans and earlier, more accurate diagnoses may result from this.

Initiatives for Policy:

Make the case for the need for laws that facilitate MG sufferers' access to vital support services, drugs, and therapies.

In essence, the conclusion ought to motivate the reader to take action in order to enhance treatment at both the individual and systemic levels and leave them with a clear understanding of the significance of a comprehensive strategy for treating myasthenia gravis.

THE END

www.ingramcontent.com/pod-product-compliance
Lightning Source LLC
Chambersburg PA
CBHW050744260726
48661CB00001B/395